IF MOMMY IS NOT HAPPY, NO ONE IS HAPPY

Pregnancy and the Injured Pelvis:
A Guide for Partners and Midwives

Dr. William J. Ruch

ISBN-13: 978-1539955696
ISBN-10: 1539955699

*This book is dedicated to the soon-to-be mother
who needs to have her baby safely
and with as little distress and pain as possible…*

*and to my mother, without whom this book
would never have been written.*

INTRODUCTION

I first met Dr. William Ruch after a back injury left me in severe pain. It was the cumulative result of more than two decades of assisting women in childbirth as a midwife. Years of twisting and turning and lifting had taken their toll on me. My daughter finally insisted I see Dr. Ruch, so off I went, expecting little. After a very gentle treatment, I hobbled back to my car and drove home, still in a fair amount of pain and disappointed. I lay down to take a nap. When I awoke, I got up and it took me a moment to realize I had no pain. I stretched, I bent, I touched my toes, I cried in relief.

I continued to see Dr. Ruch, and sent my midwife and physician colleagues to see him as well. Dr. Ruch worked with me and helped me to prevent re-injuring myself. As we talked, he explained how keeping the female pelvis aligned then in turn helped the hips, legs and back to remain stable. We talked about the ways pregnancy and childbirth change the female pelvis and can lead to mobility problems, pelvic pain and other difficulties. He then showed me some simple maneuvers to teach my clients who were experiencing pelvic, back, and hip/leg pain in pregnancy. I tried it and was so delighted to see women who had walked into my exam room obviously in pain stride out with smiles on their faces and a spring in their step.

I referred patients to Dr. Ruch when they needed more comprehensive adjustments. The feedback I got was astonishing. Women who were one step from having to stop working and at risk of being put on disability, narcotics, or had failed physical therapy were able to fully function and enjoy the rest of their pregnancies with minimal or no pain. His methodology is rooted firmly in anatomical and physiological science. It is non-invasive and it works.

I hope this will become not only part of chiropractic education, but of midwifery, osteopathic and medical education. So often the simplest seeming interventions can have the greatest impact on improving health. This is one of them that will surely make Momma happy!

Sallie P. Hill, MSN, CNM

ACKNOWLEDGEMENTS

I want to thank our model, the "mommy in red." She was very gracious and patient with us.

I want thank Zoe and Zora for helping with set up and lighting. They make working in the office a joy.

I also thank Kim Lemoine, who formatted and edited this book. This wouldn't have happened without her.

Lastly, I thank Dr. Victoria Nelson for her insights and support.

TABLE OF CONTENTS

OVERVIEW

This short handbook is for pregnant women with injuries to the pelvic girdle and those attending her before, during and after labor. It is designed to help the layperson assess and level the mother's pelvis and lessen the pain and stress of any past pelvic injury.

A QUICK ANATOMY LESSON

In the adult, the pelvic girdle is a three-bone complex including the sacrum and the right and left hip bones. Three joints unite the bones of the pelvic girdle; the two sacroiliac joints and the pubis symphysis *(see Figure 1)*.

The sacrum is the base of the spine and the pelvic girdle, as a whole, is the anchor for quite a substantial part of the muscular system of the spine, legs, thorax and abdomen. All of the abdominal, hip and thigh muscles originate from the pelvic girdle, as do the two large back muscles. So it is not difficult to see how misalignment of the pelvic girdle can affect any or all of these muscle groups, causing them to contract, become hypertonic (rigid), or go into spasm. In my clinical experience the key to understanding the cause of much "low back pain" is the loss of integrity, alignment of the three pelvic joints.

In Figures 1a and 1b some of the muscles directly involved with sacroiliac joint and pubic symphysis motion and integrity are illustrated along with the ligaments. In order for the pelvic bones to misalign, the ligaments must be failing and are injured. The muscles will then attempt to hold everything together with tightness.

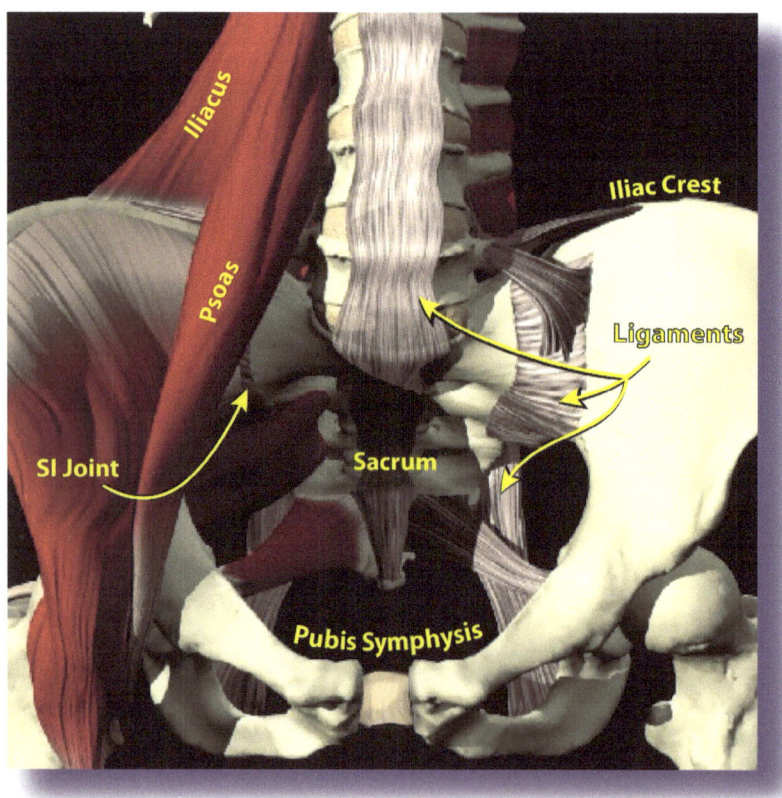

Photo printed with permission from primalpictures.com

FIGURE 1a MUSCLES AND LIGAMENTS OF THE PELVIC GIRDLE

*The **ligaments** hold the pelvic bones together. They can get injured in falls and accidents, causing misalignment.*

FIGURE 1b SIDE VIEW OF THE PELVIS

The anterior superior iliac spine or the ASIS are the front points at the end of the iliac crests

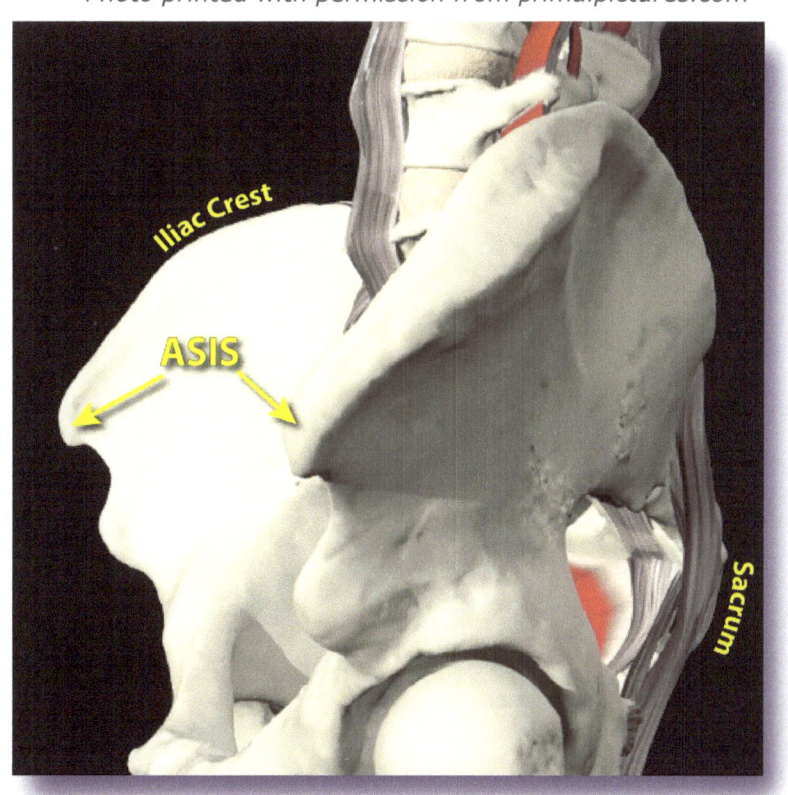

Misalignment of the Pelvis

Hip bone misalignment involves the sacroiliac (SI) joint and pubic symphysis, and will adversely affect all the deep and superficial muscles around the abdomen. The posterior muscles (back muscles and the deep hip muscles) are also affected. The psoas and iliacus muscles *(see Figure 1)* will be recruited neurologically to guard and protect the injured joints by limiting their range of motion. Misalignment can displace abdominal organs away from the origins of their nerves and arteries. Muscular distress, pain and limited range of motion will be only some of the clinical symptoms.

The Nervous System

All tissues and joints in the body are embedded with various types of sensors, or nerves. When a joint is injured or misaligned, these sensors cause muscles to "guard" or go into contraction for extended periods of time. These contractions can be quite uncomfortable. Since so many important, highly used muscles attach to the pelvis, the contractions can be extremely distressing, as the sufferer can't seem to move at all without pain. At the heart of the pelvis is the pubic symphysis. When this joint is misaligned, chaos ensues.

It is extremely important to understand that the guarding (spasmed) muscles around the pubic symphysis can, like any other muscle, be relieved *only by correcting the misalignment* and by removing nerve distress within the joint. The nervous system may never adapt to neurological input arising from joint distress—in other words, someone who suffers from joint distress will never "get used to it" as their muscles will always fire or contract if the nerves sense a misaligned joint. The common practice is to prescribe narcotics as treatment. However **drugs only mask the firing of the joint injuries**. They are a temporary solution and do not treat the cause.

Mobility and misalignment of the pelvic girdle is controversial; if it has ever happened to you, you understand how frustrating it can be to cope with the pain and confusion involved in treating such injuries. As a practicing chiropractor I encounter this type of injury every hour I am treating people. But those in the medical community, and even those in my own profession, disagree and have confusion over not only how mobility is affected by this joint but even whether misalignment of the pelvic joints occurs in the first place. The vast majority of my profession ignores the anterior joints of the body (ribs), the sternal joints (clavicle) as well as the pubic symphysis.

I am going to attempt to make this set of "re-aligning procedures" as easy for the helper and as comfortable for the patient as possible. We will be using an evaluation of the anterior (front) part of her pelvis *(see Figure 2 A)*. The figure shown is the front of the pelvis and that is the only approach we will be using. There are two bony landmarks on the front of the pelvis: the left and right Anterior Superior Iliac Spine (ASIS) and the Pubic Symphysis *(see Figures 1A and 1B).*

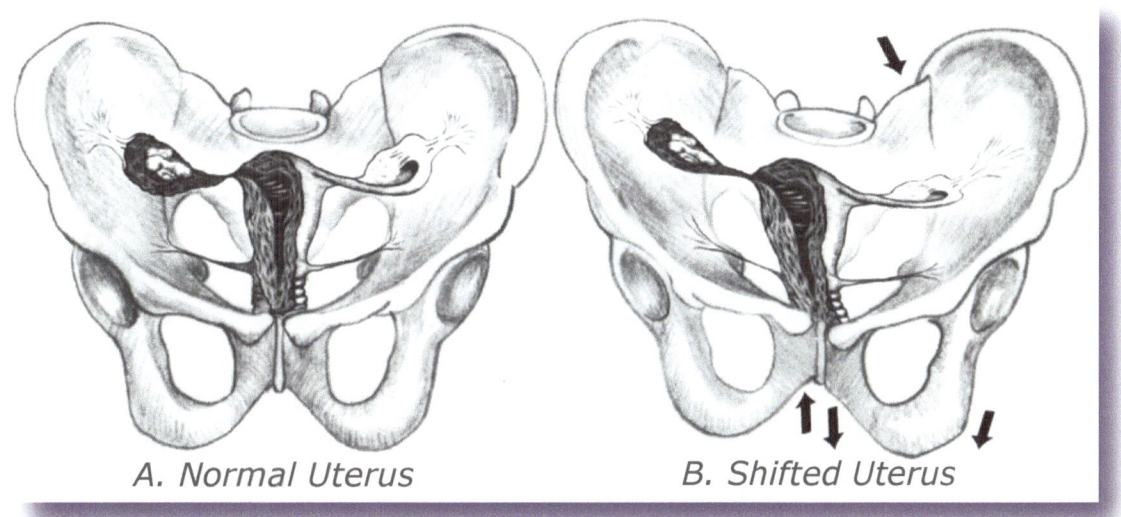

A. Normal Uterus   B. Shifted Uterus

FIGURE 2 A AND B SHIFTING OF THE UTERUS WITH PELVIC MISALIGNMENT

The uterus will shift to one side when the pelvic bones shift. This can be painful, debilitating and responsible for difficult labors.

FIGURE 3 AN X-RAY OF A MISALIGNED PELVIS WITH AIR INJECTED INTO THE UTERUS.

Note the asymmetry and the misalignment of the pubic bones and the displacement of the uterus

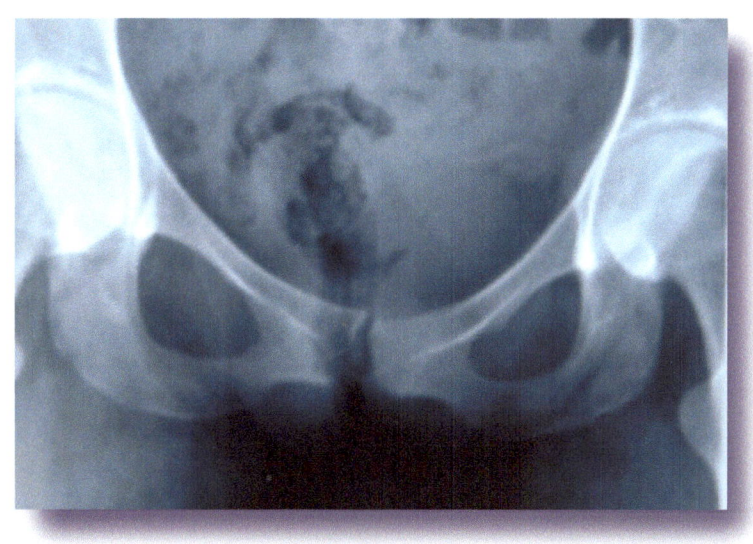

A variety of complaints can result from misalignment of the pelvic joints, including infertility, urogenital and intestinal problems. In a normal female pelvis, the broad ligament stretches between the two hip bones, suspending the ovaries and the uterus *(see Figure 2)*. When the pelvic girdle misaligns, the broad ligament becomes skewed *(see Figure 2).* This changes the position of the ovaries and the uterus in the abdominal cavity and can exacerbate any problem that might exist; the pelvic examination can reveal tight and tender musculature on one side and the uterus tractioned to one side. *(see Figure 3)*.

Note the right side shift of the gynecological structures and the pelvic misalignment. (The left side of this picture is the right side of the individual). Note misalignment of the pubic bones and the asymmetrical appearance in the lower pelvis. In late stage pregnancy, this shift, with a fetus in the uterus, will cause the fetus to "sit" or "press" on the Psoas. This will make walking difficult or impossible. This shift is responsible for some of the breech positions that occur. I think that a large percentage of gynecological pathology may be the result of unresolved pelvic trauma. Correcting misaligned pelvis has been shown clinically to relieve or reverse these conditions.

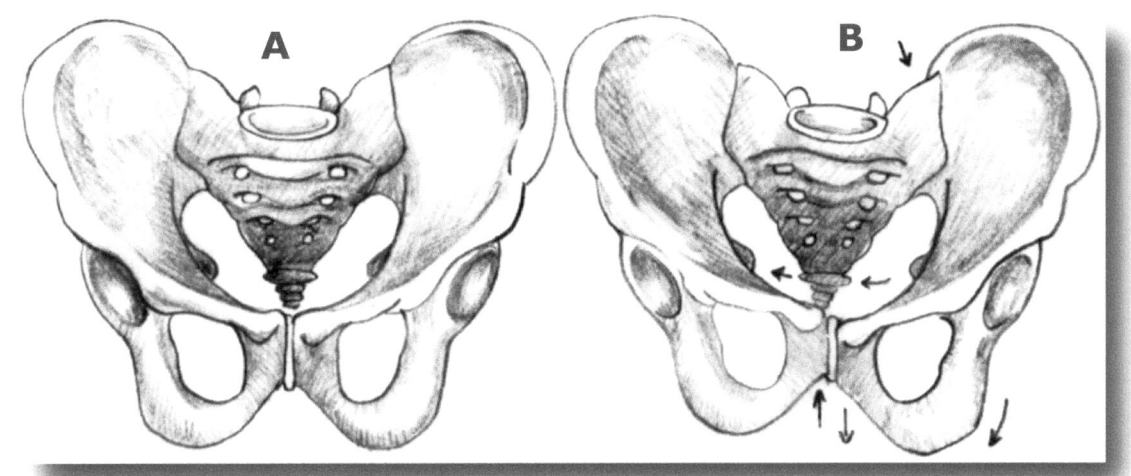

FIGURE 4 A AND B. THE SHIFT OF ONE HIP BONE UP RELATIVE TO THE OTHER

Figure 4 A shows an aligned pelvis and B is the "up slipped" hipbone. Note the misalignment involves the ASIS and crest of each bone, not just the pubic symphysis.

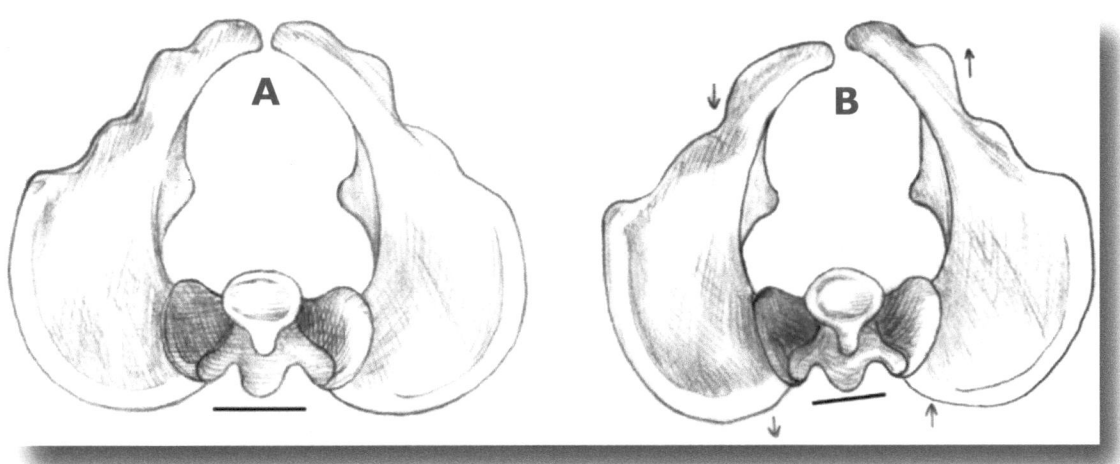

FIGURE 5 A AND B. THE FORWARD SHIFT OF ONE HIP BONE TO THE OTHER.

In figure 5 A the pelvis is aligned. In figure 5 B the right hipbone is forward of the other. This can be felt by touching the front of the pelvis (see figure 11).

Pregnancy and the pelvis require special attention if there has been a previous history of injury to the pelvic joints. This protocol is appropriate for late stage pregnancy when distress patterns can be significant, but can be used throughout the pregnancy. The significant displacement of the pubic bones relative to each other is a major pain producing factor. *(see Figures 4 A and B on the preceding page).* **Evaluating the pattern of misalignment is critical.**

START WITH AN ASSESSMENT

Place the mom in a supine (face up) tilted up posture *(see Figure 6).* Have the mom find her ASIS on each side *(see Figure 7).* Note any asymmetry and tenderness. The helper should verify the findings *(see Figure 8)*. Then have the patient find her pubic symphysis, if she can. She may not be able to reach it. In any case the helper should palpate the pubic symphysis by starting at the ASIS on each side and sweeping the palpating fingers underneath the abdomen until they reach the midline. If there is any sensitivity or pain then the pubic symphysis is likely misaligned, especially if asymmetry at the ASIS is noted *(see Figure 9).*

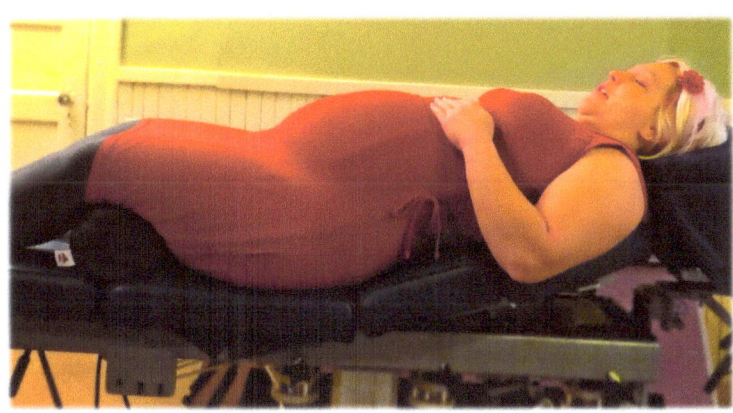

Figure 6 SUPINE POSITION

This is usually the most comfortable position for Mom instead of flat on her back.

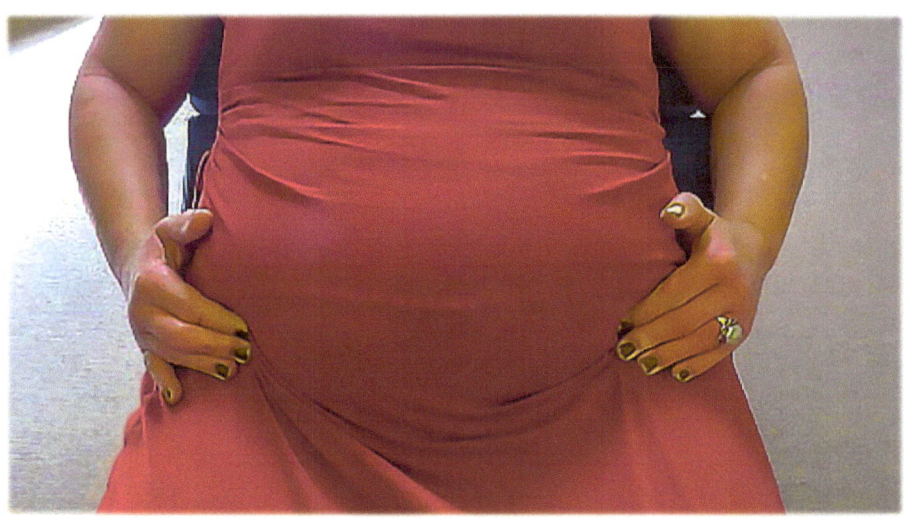

Figure 7 THE MOM FINDS HER ANTERIOR SUPERIOR ILIAC SPINE (ASIS) ON EACH SIDE

Have the mom put her fingers on her ASIS on each side and note any asymmetry in height and posteriority. This mom's left ASIS is superior and posterior relative to the right side.

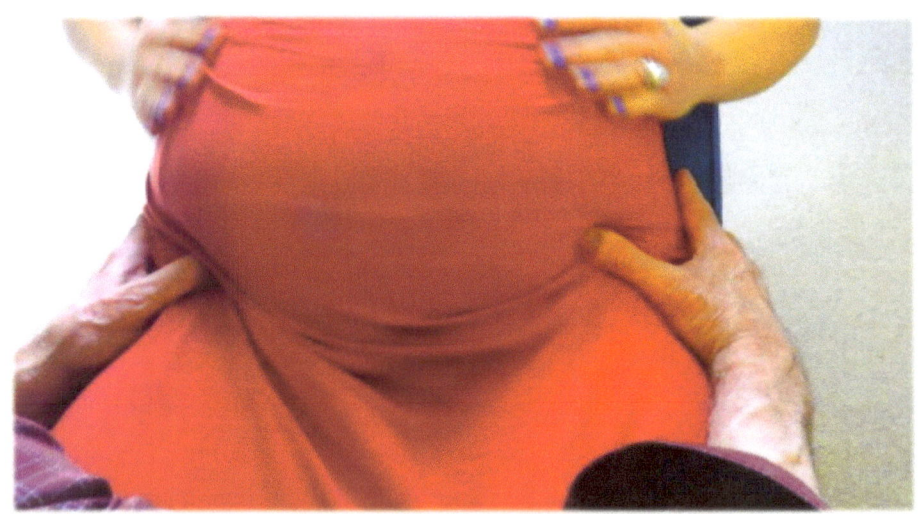

Figure 8 THE HELPER VERIFIES THE POSITIONS OF THE ASIS ON EACH SIDE.

The helper's thumbs are on the ASIS on each side to verify that the left ASIS is superior (higher) and posterior (further back) compared to the right side.

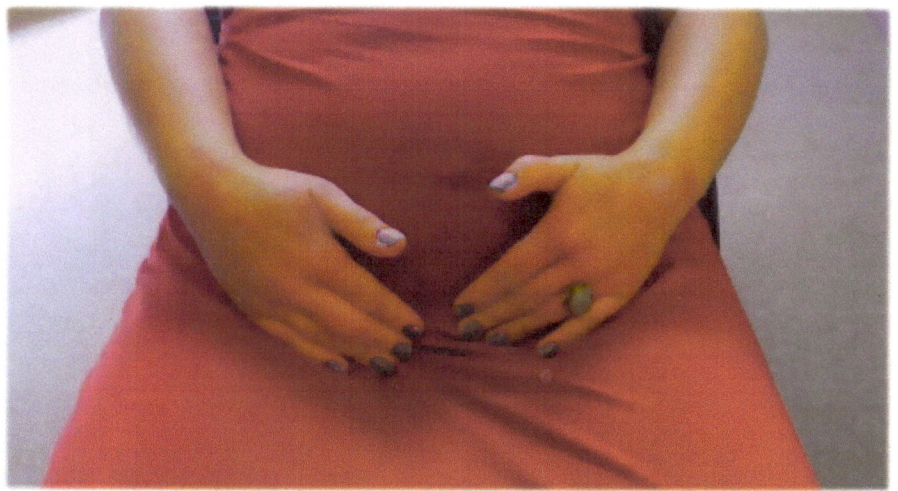

Figure 9 THE MOM CONTACTS HER PUBIC SYMPHYSIS, ANTERIOR SURFACE

This mom has significant pain at the pubic symphysis. Note the posterior or backward position of her left hand.

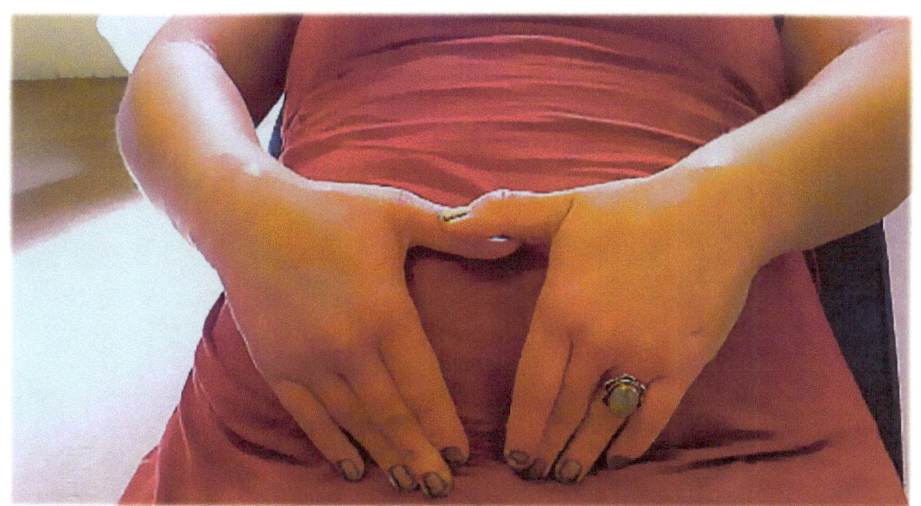

Figure 10 THE MOM CONTACTS HER PUBIC SYMPHYSIS ON THE SUPERIOR (HIGHER) SURFACE

The superior displacement of the hip bone is the most painful and debilitating of the displacement patterns.

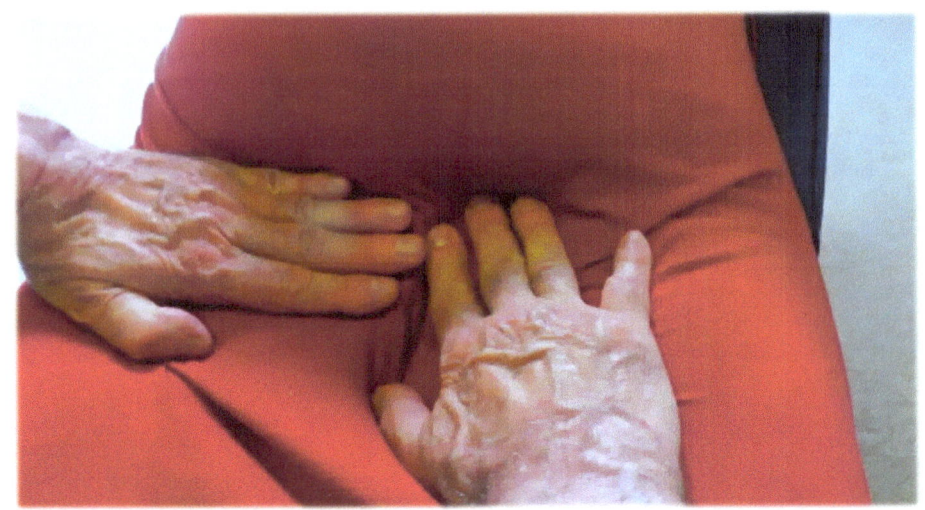

Figure 11 THE HELPER'S HANDS ON THE ANTERIOR PUBIC SYMPHSIS

*The helper's hands palpate (feel or touch) the anterior surface of the pubic bones. Sometimes the mom is so big she cannot feel her own pubic bones. The helper should do this and note misalignment and pain. **Reduction of misalignment and pain are the goals.***

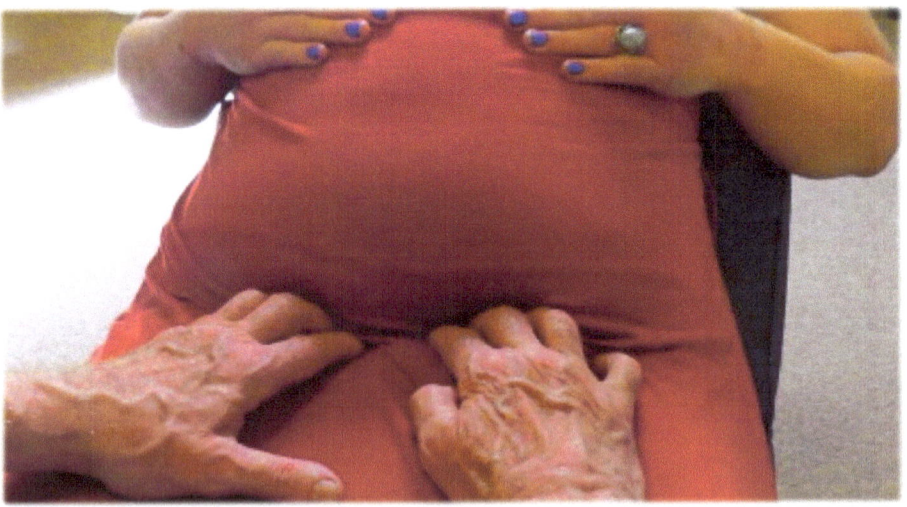

Figure 12 THE HELPER'S HANDS ON THE SUPERIOR PUBIC BONES

The helper's fingers palpate the top of the pubic bones evaluating the misalignment pattern. Note the hand on the patients left side is more superior.

The maneuvers are focused on reducing or eliminating pain at the pubic symphysis by realigning the pubic bones. If there is tenderness and pain, you need to note the posterior or backward side of the two bones and then a higher or more superior ASIS of the pair. Have the mom contact the top of her pubic bones, see Figure 10. The helper might have to verify the misalignment pattern, see Figure 11.

MANEUVERS FOR RE-ALIGNMENT

Leg Pull/Hip Bone Push

The high or superior side will be the side for the leg pull. The mom will have her other leg straight against the helper's thigh *(see Figure 13)*. The mom's foot is up against the helper's thigh, the helper has a hold of the opposite leg at the top of the calf (just below the knee) and around the ankle. This process is done slowly, repetitively and firmly with the response of the mom noted.

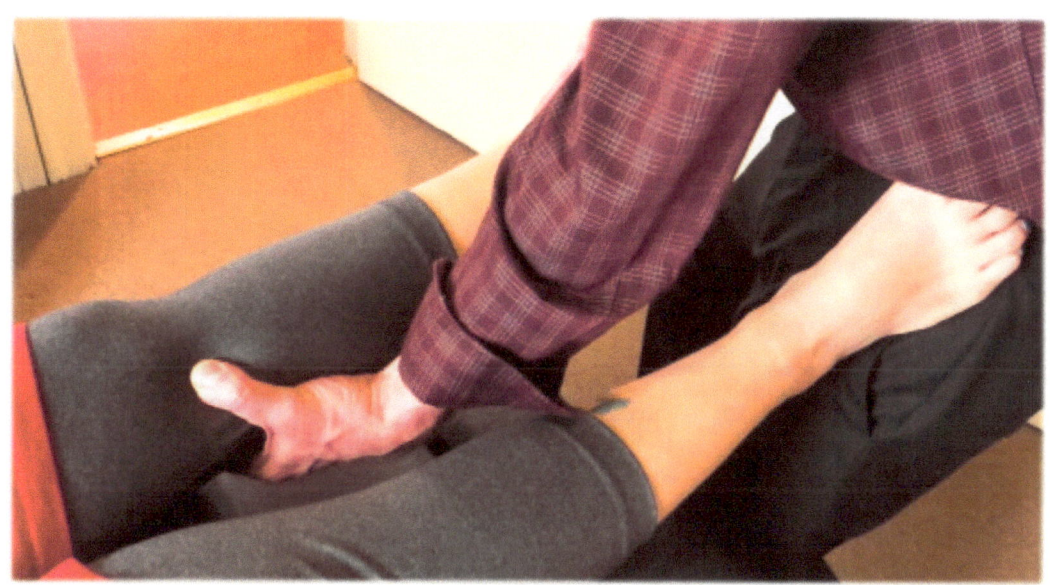

Figure 13 PERFORMING THE LEG PULL

Performing this maneuver many times rather than all at once allows reduced forces. This procedure is done until the top of the pubic bones are level and the pain is gone.

An alternative to the leg pull is the hip bone pushing *(see Figure 14)*. The helper contacts the iliac crest and the top of the leg bone. The pushing is towards the feet. Pushing the hip bone might have to be done during active labor if the leg pulling is not comfortable or not feasible.

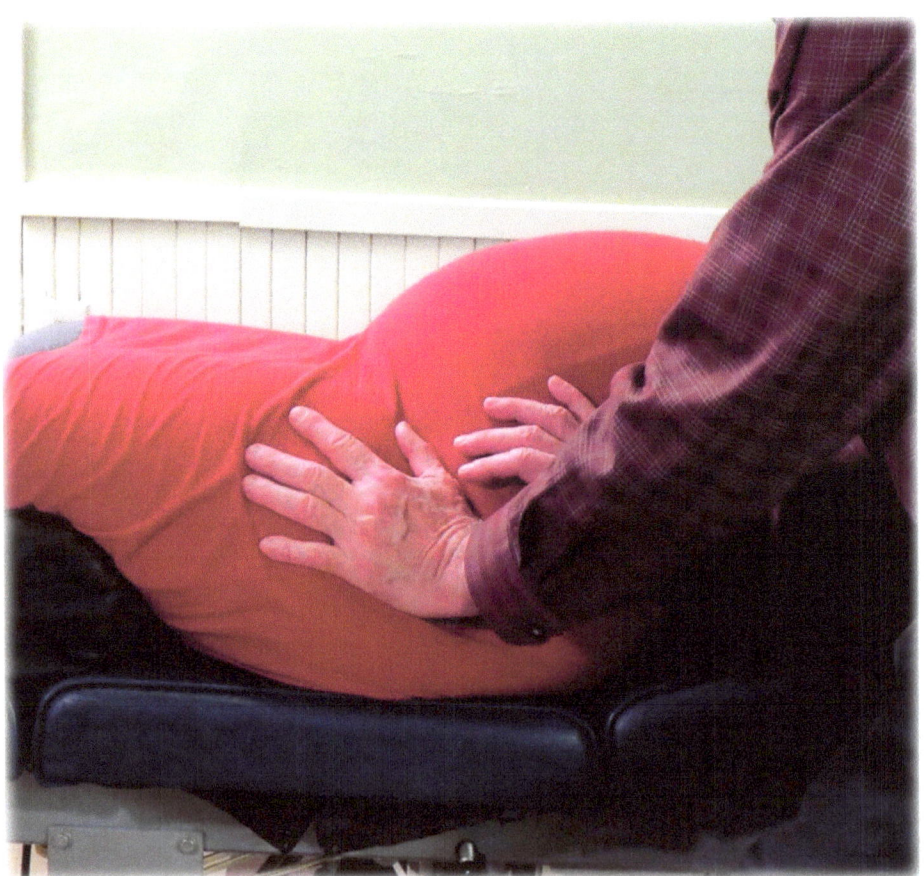

Figure 14 HIP BONE PUSHING
The helper is contacting the top of the crest of the hip bone and the top of the leg bone, pushing downwards towards the feet.

The Backward Push

The forward side will have a small firm pillow or foam wedge placed underneath the **opposite** side *(see Figure 15)*. The helper's hands are placed on the thigh and hip of the forward side and gently pushed towards the table or posteriorly at an angle towards the midline of the mom *(see Figure 16)*.

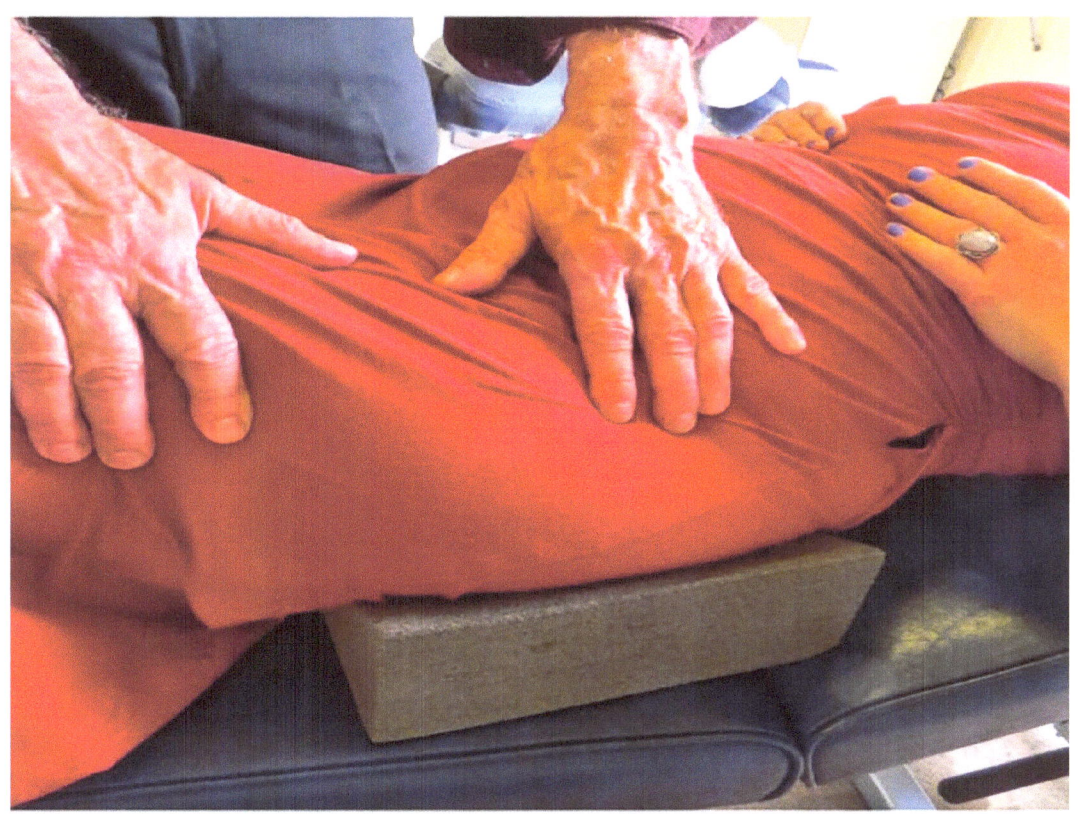

Figure 15 SETTING UP THE BACKWARD PUSH
The mom will have a cushion or support under the posterior or backward side

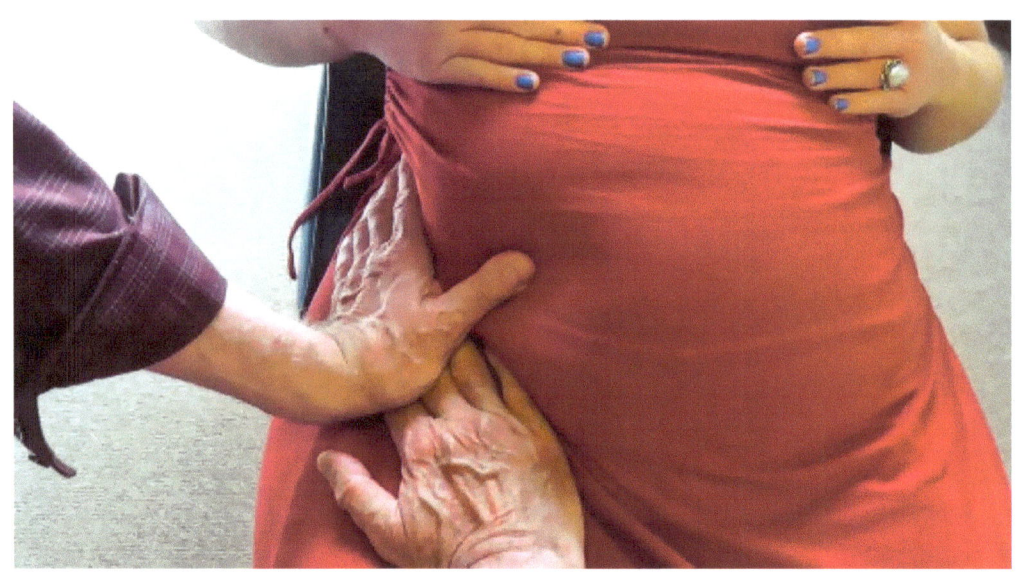

Figure 16 PERFORMING THE BACKWARD PUSH

Gentle, repetitive thrusts are done on the side that is forward towards the mom's back at an angle towards the midline.

RE-EVALUATE

Both the leg pulling and the backward pushing are done until an evaluation of the pubic symphysis is painless and level *(see Figure 17)*. Please compare Figure 10 to Figure 20. I admit this can be pretty subtle, especially as care proceeds. Tenderness and limited motion are indications of guarding patterns from joint distress.

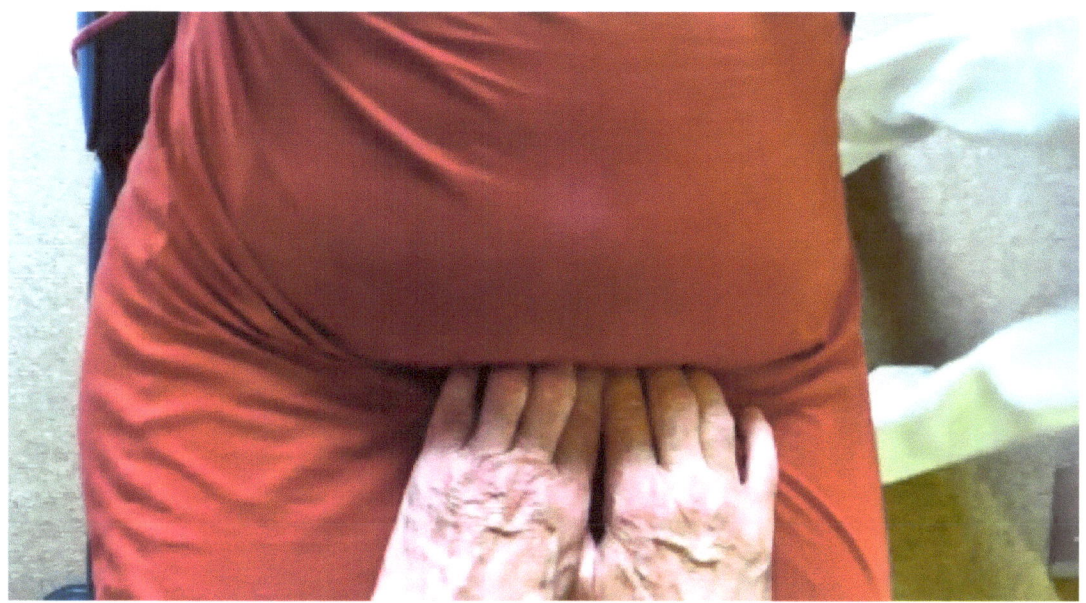

Figure 17 RE-EVALUATING, POST LEVELING

The aligned pubic bones. The helper's hands go over an aligned, smooth, non-tender joint.

The goal here is that the pubic bones are aligned. Be thorough; get rid of as much pain as possible. We need "dead level" at both the top and front components of the pubic bones. In this view the patient is being evaluated for front to back or anterior-posterior misalignment. This shows an aligned pubic symphysis, with no tenderness-- a big difference from her presenting condition.

This is critical; the slipping up of the hipbone is the most painful of the misalignment patterns. When the pubic bones are level across the top there is a relaxation of the abdominal wall. Also, the mother can often feel the baby shifting back to the midline. In this view we have a level pubic symphysis and no pain.

This patient's pattern here was high on the left. A recent Ultrasound showed the baby all pulled over the left side. Upon leveling her pelvis, she felt the baby shift to the middle of her abdomen.

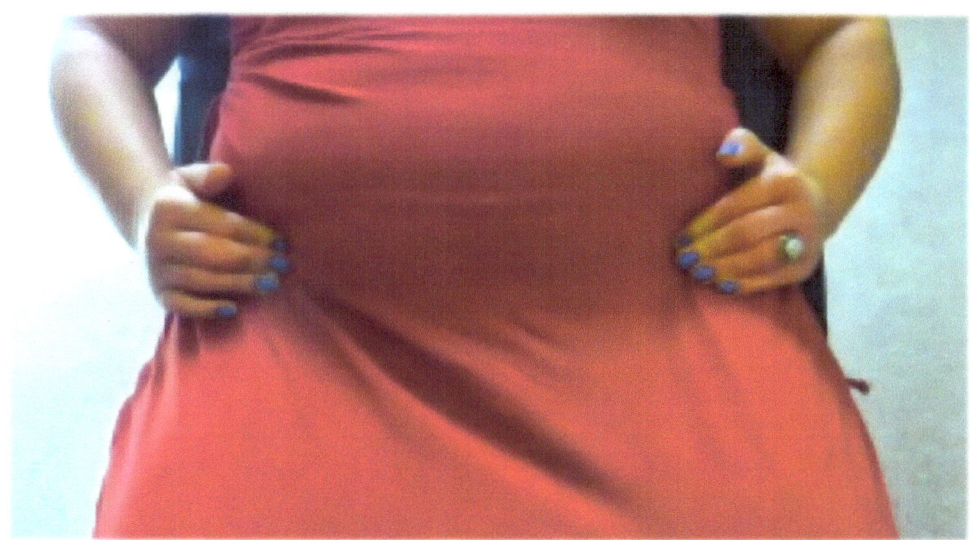

Figure 18
RE-EVALUATING THE HIGH OR SUPERIOR SIDE
The ASIS alignment looks good. Compare this to Figure 7 and 8 below

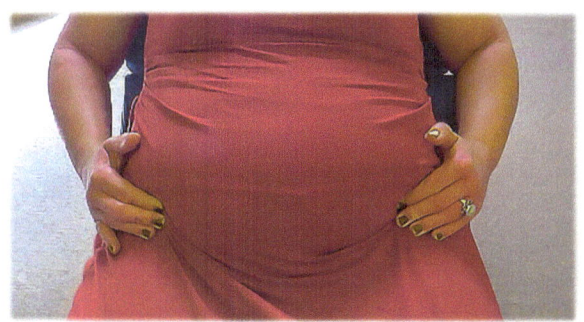 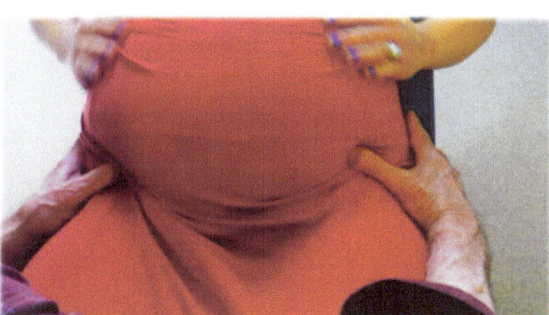

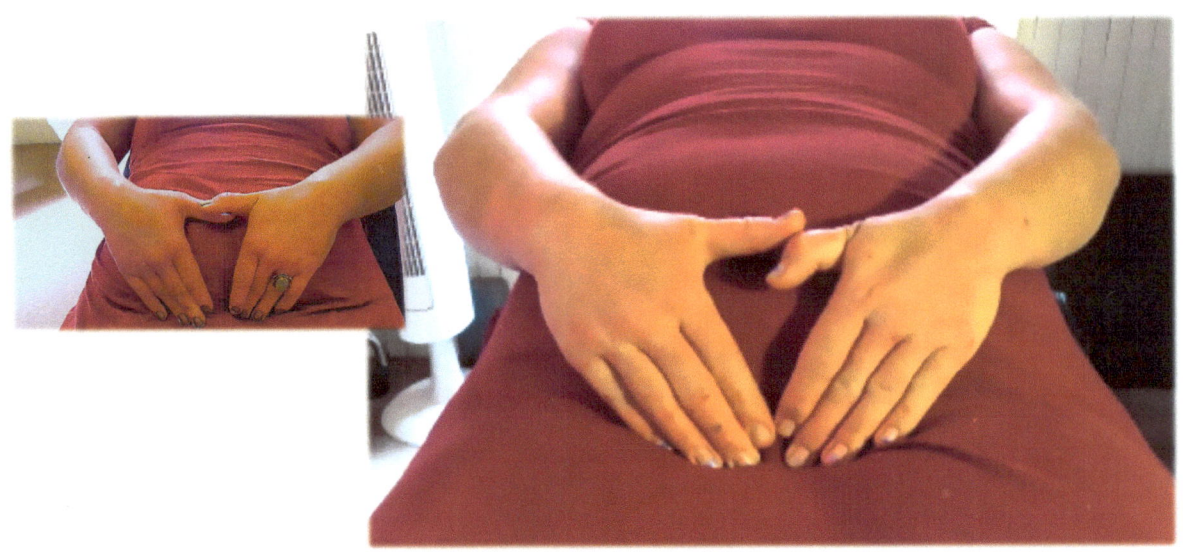

**Figure 19 SELF RE-EVALUATION
OF THE ANTERIOR PUBIC SYMPHYSIS**

The patient can contact the anterior surface of her pubic symphysis for tenderness or pain and signs of misalignment. There is no pain at this point for the mom. Compare this to Figure 9, above left.

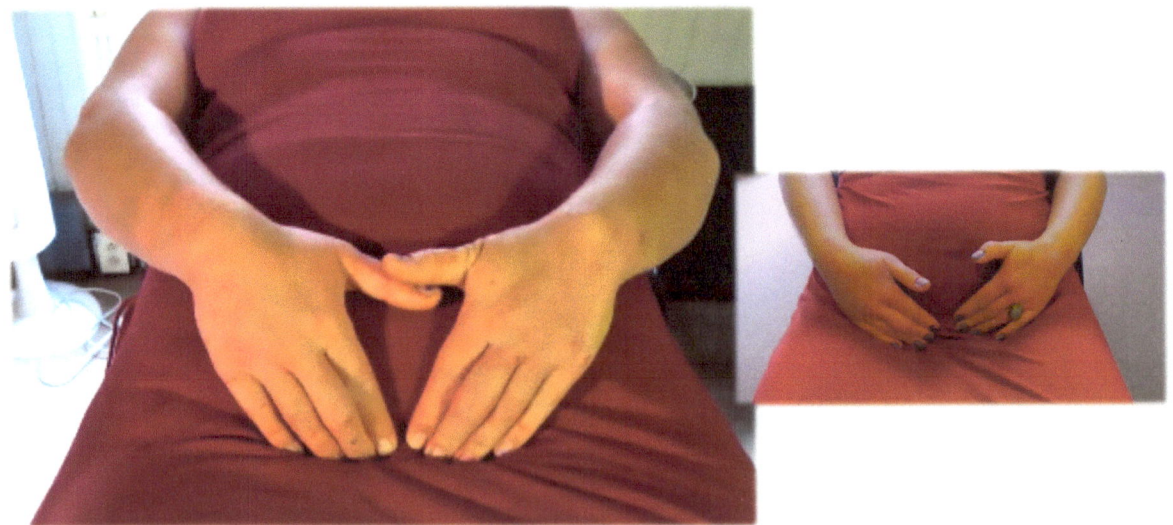

**Figure 20 SELF RE-EVALUATION
OF THE SUPERIOR PUBIC SYMPHYSIS**

This mom can self-evaluate the superior displacement of her pubic symphysis, though she might not be able to do this in late stage pregnancy. Compare this to Figure 10, above right.

MANAGEMENT OF PREGNANT PELVIS

The pattern for a majority of women with problems of pain and mobility during pregnancy is that the high side (as determined by supine evaluation) will have the uterus, and therefore the baby, shifts to that side. Depending on pelvic tilt, the shift could put the fetus into contact with the Psoas. This muscle lifts the leg. Some mothers will have a hard time walking and standing.

The mom can be taught how to do self-evaluation and monitor her behavior and resulting misalignment patterns. The pictured patient has two small children and is pregnant with her third. There are lots of ways for her to get hurt. The goals we have with these protocols are multiple.

1. We want the partner, or whoever is helping, to be doing the leg pulling and the backwards pushing to keep the pelvis level. One main reason is to benefit the mother. She needs to have her usual ability to walk around with minimal pain. Here is the universal rule that **if mommy is not happy no one's happy.**

2. We want the baby to be comfortable, experiencing the needed movement of mother walking around and being active. The baby thrives when this is happening, and when the mother is distressed, the baby is distressed.

3. We need the partner to know how to keep the mom's pelvis level, not only through the remainder of her pregnancy, but through labor and delivery as well.

I feel most of the difficulties in labor and delivery are due to the maternal un-level or misaligned pelvis. We know that the un-level pelvis and its relationship to labor and delivery is not understood by the midwives and the OB/GYN's. Our experience is that for a lot of our patients, when the pelvis is level at delivery, things can go pretty quickly.

We recommend the pelvic leveling take place three times a day, if possible: First thing in the morning, midday or as early in the evening as possible, and then at bedtime. As a general rule, in the third trimester, I recommend avoiding sitting on soft couches or the floor, or anywhere where you sink into something or have to twist and climb to get on your feet. This could mean the bathtub has to be given up. This is managing an unstable pelvis, so modifications of personal behavior have to take place. It's much better for the patient to sit or be perched on a stool or take the cushions off the couch and put them on the kitchen chair so her hips are boosted above her knees. This is especially important if the patient is also suffering from wrist hand and shoulder injuries. Pushing and managing her position changes in the advanced pregnant state is a factor that can create additional injuries in the upper body.

Pelvic instability, if pre-pregnancy, could be a lifetime problem. Note the presence of the relaxin hormone will be influencing the pelvic stability for weeks or months post-delivery. This period of time gets longer with each pregnancy. The additional work of baby care followed by childcare can set the patient up for chronic pain.

A STORY

A few years ago my daughter Rachel arrived at the house we rent at the beach and she could not get out of the car without help. She was due in four days. She could barely stand or walk. As she started for the front door, I directed her to the sidewalk alongside the side of the house and to the deck in the back where a chiropractic table was ready for her. She needed help to get to the table. We placed her in the supine tilted position, *(see Figure 6)*. I then evaluated her and asked her partner, Randall, to reconfirm my evaluation. Rachel was in severe distress and the pubic symphysis was significantly misaligned. Palpation of the ASIS's showed that she was high on the left side and palpation of the pubic symphysis showed that she was anterior on the right side. I then showed Randall how to do the leg pull on her left side and the backwards push on her right side. He repeated each maneuver 5 to 6 times, then rechecked the pubic symphysis until there was no tenderness and the bones were aligned anteriorly (front) and superiorly (up). The ASIS's were level. We then had her roll onto her right side to sit up. Note that she was high on the left side and we do not want her loading that left side with changing positions or lifting things. **This is a major management issue.** At that moment Rachel was able to stand up and walk around without distress. She did a few deep knee bends, she declared herself fine and then they went for a walk on the beach. I had Randall practice a few more times through the weekend. Tuesday morning she went into labor and delivered in eight hours. She had a natural childbirth without complications. When I arrived shortly after, I was told that Randall was a great help to Rachel.

In just about five minutes of instruction and a few practice sessions, Randall was able to learn these simple techniques, saving Rachel much pain and discomfort before, during and after her labor.

ANOTHER STORY

"Gina" came to our office in January of 2015. She was primarily complaining of right ankle, foot and leg pain. She had the additional complaint of chronic low back pain, very painful monthly periods, losing 4 to 6 days of work per month due to heavy bleeding and pain. Also she said that at age 13 (she is now 34) she was told she had a bifurcated uterus and could never conceive. She had just finished adopting her second child, who was 1 year old and she had already adopted a 3½ year old. We started care with her, addressing all the issues, including leveling the pelvis. Her pubic bones were significantly tender and un-level. In April she told me her "period pain" had diminished significantly. In June she said her period was pain free, including her chronic low back pain. In August she came into the office, stopped in the doorway to the treatment area and announced:

"Dr. Ruch I am pregnant and it's all your fault!"
Danielle was born in March of 2016.

These maneuvers can be used to keep the mother happy, but also can be used to manage chronic low back pain, painful periods and infertility.

ABOUT THE AUTHOR

Dr. William Ruch has run a full-time private practice of chiropractic for thirty years. He got his Bachelor of Science degree in Biology from the University of San Francisco in 1975, and graduated Cum Laude from Life Chiropractic College West in Hayward, California in September of 1986. Dr. Ruch has authored multiple scientific articles that have appeared in chiropractic journals. He has also authored a textbook/atlas on spinal and pelvic pathophysiology, including cadaver dissection study photographs and radiology. In addition, he has authored chapters on the autonomic neuroanatomy of the vertebral subluxation/misalignment complex, published several cadaver specimens and radiograph photography in other textbooks, developed numerous slide and video presentations, and has even invented and patented medical device for carpal tunnel syndrome and other repetitive stress disorders.